Health Care at Home
A Family Massage Manual

Chen Zhaoguang

Foreign Languages Press   Beijing

First Edition 1992
Second Printing 1997

Illustrated by Li Shiji
Translated by Zhao Yong

ISBN 7-119-01480-3

© Foreign Languages Press, Beijing, China, 1992

Published by Foreign Languages Press
24 Baiwanzhuang Road, Beijing 100037, China

Distributed by China International Book Trading Corporation
35 Chegongzhuang Xilu, Beijing 100044, China
P.O. Box 399, Beijing, China

Printed in the People's Republic of China

Contents

Introduction 1
What is *yin-yang*?
What is *qi*?
What are meridians and collaterals?
What is "general acupoint massage"?
Why is it good?
Indications and Contraindications
Notes and Cautions
How long is one *cun*?

Questions and Answers 9
1. Why does this massage start from the foot?
2. If I want to treat a particular disease, what shall I do?
3. How frequently and how long am I supposed to do this massage?
4. Why are there "transient manipulations"?
5. Why in some steps am I supposed to tap randomly at a certain place?

Manipulations 12
Category 1: Manipulations That Promote the Circulation of Qi and Blood
Category 2: Manipulations Smoothing the Meridians and Collaterals

Acupoints Used in This Massage 21
Massage Operation 1: Massage for Two People 23
Massage Operation 2: Self-Massage 107
Indices 138

Introduction

For the over one billion Chinese people, massage, acupuncture, moxibustion and herbal medicine are familiar and trusted methods of health care. Across China, there are nearly 300,000 doctors practicing Chinese medicine and nearly 2,000 hospitals specializing in Chinese medicine, not to mention that almost in every general hospital there is a section where the patients are treated with traditional Chinese medical methods. A more astounding fact is that the people of China, despite their low living standard, have an average lifespan of sixty-nine. In this regard, Chinese medicine with traditional methods of health care certainly plays an important role.

This is a fact of daily life, with no mystery about it. On the other hand, Chinese medicine was founded on the basis of ancient Chinese philosophy which is quite alien to the thinking of people from other cultures. Thus, it is appropriate to first examine some basic concepts commonly used in Chinese medicine.

What is *yin-yang*?

Yin-yang is the basic classification of the material world in ancient Chinese thought. Everything can be assigned to either *yin* or *yang*. *Yang* pertains to masculine, strong, positive, upward properties, while *yin* pertains to feminine, weak, negative, downward properties.

They are ever opposing, but also complementing each other, the existence of either one being the prerequisite of the other. Without *yin*, there would be no *yang*; and without *yang*, there would be no *yin*.

Yin-yang is also a basic element of traditional Chinese medical theories. It is used to explain the integrated, organic structure of the human body, its physiological functions and pathological changes.

What is *qi*?

Literally, *qi* means air. Philosophically, *qi* is the prime element of the universe, according to the ancient thought. It is the changes and movement of *qi* that produce all the phenomena of the universe. In theories of Chinese medicine, which is greatly influenced by ancient thought, *qi* can be translated as "life force." *Qi* within the human body is invisible, but it is manifested by the functions of the body organs.

Qi extends to all parts of the body and determines every part's well-being. Abundance of *qi* is the basis of good health and weakness of *qi* may lead to diseases.

There is a close relationship between *qi* and blood.

What are meridians and collaterals?

Briefly, meridians and collaterals are the passages through which *qi* and blood circulates. In an extensive network, they cover the entire body, interior and exterior. They transport *qi* and blood, regulate *yin* and *yang* of the human body, and adjust physiological balance.

According to Chinese medical theory, pathogenic factors come from two sources: from the human body itself, particularly emotions (such as joy, anger, melancholy, worry, grief, fear, and fright) and from the natural world, particularly the atmospheric changes (such as wind, cold, dryness, summer heat and humidity), together with improper diet and living habits. When a certain organ is impaired by pathogenic factors, it fails to function well. Moreover, as meridians and collaterals reach every part of the body and are connected with each other, the sick organ may send negative information to other organs through the meridians and collaterals, resulting in another sick organ. For example, cirrhosis of the liver may lead to splenomegaly, pulmonary emphysema may be complicated with pulmonary heart disease.

Along the meridians and collaterals there are points called acupoints. They are the sites where the *qi* of body organs and meridians reach the body surface. Different points relate to different organs and meridians. So acupoints are the place where we can "talk" with the body and its organs.

From this review, we can see that acupoints are the windows of the body. Furthermore, when pathological changes develop in visceral organs, there are sensations of pain, tingling, etc., at the corresponding acupoints, or round- or bar-shaped scleromata, or bigger areas that are highly sensitive to pressure. This is the result of the information of the diseased visceral organ being carried out to the body surface through the meridians. In turn, if we feed information back through the acupoints, the corresponding organ will respond. The information feedback is actually the massage, acupuncture and moxibustion applied to the acupoints. For example, patients with gastric diseases feel pain on Zusanli (ST 36) point when it is pressed. Massage on Zusanli (ST 36) will make the patient feel relieved and comfortable.

What is "general acupoint massage"?

"General acupoint massage" is a set of massage all over the body created according to long-term clinical experience and research into massage treatment. Among the large number of acupoints, the most effective ones are selected and used in coordination. Starting from the feet, moving along the meridians, to the head, the back, and returning to the feet, massage manipulations such as digital pressing, fingertip tapping and hand rolling activate the acupoints, making all parts of the body coherent and in connection with each other through a system of acupoints. This improves the body's power of resistance to unhealthy external influences and leads to timely recovery of the ailing parts.

At first we used this massage as a supplementary treatment for patients convalescent from apoplectic hemiplegia and cardiovascular diseases. Later we performed this massage regularly on patients with serious kidney disease and diabetes unresponsive to medicines. It has proved to be very effective. While experiencing success over diseases of visceral organs and the circulatory system, we also have found the massage suitable to many other diseases such as scapulohumeral periarthritis, lumbar muscle strain, sciatica, and cervical spondylopathy.

Why is it good?

"General acupoint massage," unlike common massage methods which concentrate on a particular disease, emphasizes the concept of viewing and treating the body parts as a whole, approaching a problem from various perspectives, and regarding any problem as a problem of the whole body. So this set of massage is formulated primarily to improve the general condition. At the same time, it is particularly effective in curing visceral diseases.

This massage can be done without any equipment and under almost any conditions, so it is easily used as a way of home health care between husband and wife, or between family members. For old people, the capacity of the heart and lungs declines, resulting in a shortage of *qi* and blood. This causes failure of functional coordination among the visceral organs and malnutrition. Under such conditions, old people tend to contract diseases. To ward off this danger, medicines and tonics alone are not enough, because they can't help the organs to improve themselves. This massage, however, can improve health by strengthening the positive *qi* and therefore nourishing the blood. It can effectively prevent diseases in the old such as headache and vertigo due to cerebral ischemia and senile dementia.

In the course of the massage, insidious diseases can also be detected in the light of their reflection on the superficies. Thus, the diseases can be treated at an early stage.

The massage is also good for the operator. During the course of the massage, the operator has to consume a certain amount of energy, activating the body organs to a higher level of activity and increasing metabolism. It is indeed an exercise for the visceral organs and the limbs. Therefore, this can be regarded as an exercise therapy.

Note: Although the effect of this massage is clinically proved, patients with serious diseases should not be treated solely with the massage, because it is not formulated for the treatment of any particular condition. In these cases, it is advised to use the massage as a supplement to the doctor's treatment and an excercise at home for improving health condition.

Indications and Contraindications
(Indications)
Nephritis, pyelonephritis, diabetes, myocardial ischemia, gastric diseases, diseases of the circulatory system, hemiplegia, facial paralysis, sciatica, nervous headaches, myasthenia, spinal arachnoiditis, impotence, premature ejaculation, irregular menstruation, infantile dyspepsia, stiff neck, scapulohumeral periarthritis, cervical spondylosis, protrusion of the intervertebral disc, acute lumbar muscle sprain, cervicodynia, scapulalgia, lumbago, scelalgia, rheumatism, rheumatoid arthritis, angitis, neurasthenia, climacteric syndrome, dyshormonism, apoplexy, senile aseptic necrosis of head of femur, influenza.
(Contraindications)
Acute inflammations such as suppurative tonsillitis; acute abdomen such as appendicitis, gastric and duodenal perforation; febrile disease, infectious diseases; diseases with bleeding tendency, such as thrombocytopenia, hemophilia, purpura; serious skin diseases. Warning: this massage must not be performed on pregnant women.

Notes and Cautions
The operator's fingernails should be cut short. The operator should concentrate his/her attention when doing the massage. Avoid harsh, abrupt and too heavy manipulations. For patients with heart disease or hyper-

tension, manipulation should begin with moderate force and gradually get to normal operation.

The massage is not supposed to be practiced within two hours after a meal. Keep the room appropriately warm. Never manipulate with cool hands—rub them together to warm them up before massaging.

It takes 45 to 60 minutes to complete either of the two sets of massage. After the massage, both the operator and the patient should drink a cup of water.

Don't miss points. Except those on the anterior and posterior midlines of the body, all acupoints are symmetrically in pairs on the left and right sides from the midlines.

If the *Pinyin* names of the acupoints are hard to come by, take the alphameric codes in the brackets.

How long is one *cun*?

When locating the acupoints, besides using the body's landmarks such as the five sense organs, hairlines, nails, nipples, umbilicus, prominences and depressions of bones, creases on the skin, etc., the unit of *cun* (pro-

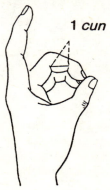

1 *cun*

nounced tsuen) is usually used.

There are several means to measure *cun*. When the middle finger of the person who receives the massage is flexed, the distance between the two medial ends of the creases of the interphalangeal joints is taken as one *cun*. Also, the width of the interphalangeal joint of the patient's thumb is taken as one *cun*. The width of the four (index, middle, ring and little) fingers close together at the level of the dorsal skin crease of the proximal interphalangeal joint of the middle finger is taken as three *cun*.

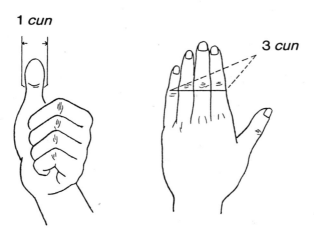

Questions and Answers

1. Why does this massage start from the foot?
Answer: Usually, the order is from the head to the foot. But the foot is the "end of the body," far from the visceral organs, where blood circulation is relatively slow. Local stagnancy of *qi* and blood tends to happen in the foot and affect the general circulation of *qi* and blood of the whole body. Starting from the foot can give a warming-up effect to the body so that the whole process will go smoothly. Besides, some pathological changes of visceral organs are reflected on the sole: there may be a lump or feeling of pain on a certain region. Sometimes, the sole is called "the second heart".

2. If I want to treat a particular disease, what shall I do?
Answer: Massage on a few selected points is permitted, but we propose that the whole set of massages be done first. Even in treating a particular disease, we believe, it is better to activate the whole organism first before massaging those acupoints which indicate that disease particularly. Again, we warn you not to depend solely on the massage for cure, although in some cases it has been as powerful as that.

3. How frequently and how long am I supposed to do this massage?

Answer: You can do it as often as once a day. For treating a disease, the minimum is two to three times each week for a total of 30 times as a course. Pause for half a month. Then start another course. This is quite effective for some chronic diseases. After the courses, doing it once or twice a week over a long term will prevent recurrence.

For those who just want to improve their health, perform the massage at least once a week. For people interested in athletic achievement, this massage is very good for relaxing and balancing functions of the body organs.

4. Why are there "transient manipulations"?

Answer: In short, transient manipulations are designed to connect different steps and make the whole process coherent. They are mostly applied to larger areas along the meridians. They have an effect of balancing the force of successive manipulations. Sometimes, it is not enough to massage the acupoint alone. For example, gastrosis makes not only Zusanli (ST 36) point painful to pressure but larger areas around the point. Transient manipulations cover such kind of areas.

5. Why in some steps am I supposed to tap randomly at a certain place?

Answer: Random tapping with varying force and speed is used to stir and smooth the meridians. You can try an experiment: tap Yiming (EX-HN 14) on the head, and you will feel a pulse corresponding to the tapping at Taichong (LR 3) on the foot. Different parts of the body are connected and must be connected. The random tapping smooths the meridians so that *qi* and blood can circulate freely. Random tapping has a better effect than tapping at a regular rhythm, because under a regular rhythm the body is prepared to receive the tapping and develops a kind of resistance. If people get hit unprepared, they always feel more pain than otherwise. For the random tapping, it is the same dynamic. It stirs up the body more.

Manipulations

Manipulations used in this massage can be classified into two categories: those promoting the circulation of *qi* and blood and those smoothing the meridians and collaterals. There are eight main methods, each with a few variations.

Category 1: Manipulations That Promote the Circulation of Qi and Blood

1. Hand Rolling
There are two ways of hand rolling. For the first, with the fingers and thumb relaxed, roll the dorsum of the hand over the patient's body—this is often applied to the old and weak (Fig. 1-1). An alternative is to clench a fist and take the wrist with the other hand to add force while rolling the fist on the patient (Fig. 1-2). This fist rolling is suitable for relatively strong people. Hand rolling is often performed on the back and chest. The track of hand rolling is usually in three forms (Fig. 1-3).

2. Rubbing
Rubbing can be performed with the palm, elbow, thumb or finger. For palm rubbing, use the heel of the hand, moving it to the left and right (Fig. 1-4). Its moving track is the same as that of hand rolling. It is

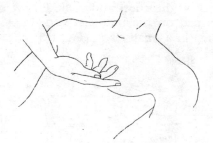

Fig. 1-1

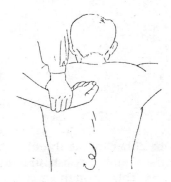

Fig. 1-2

Fig. 1-3

often applied on the chest and back Elbow rubbing is often performed on the buttocks and limbs, with the elbow moving in a small circle (Fig. 1-5).

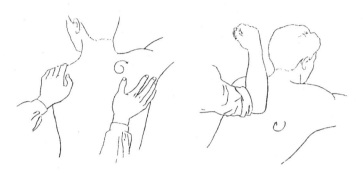

Fig. 1-4   Fig. 1-5

3. Pushing

Pushing is done either by the thumb or by the palm. With force, use the thumb to push straight ahead or at an angle (Fig. 1-6). This is often used on the muscles lateral to the vertebrae, or on the costal fovea or the route of a meridian. For palm pushing, the force comes from the heel of the hand (Fig. 1-7).

4. Grasping

There are three methods. Grasp the designated place and lift it for a while with the right and left hands in turn (Fig. 1-8). This is usually done on the limbs. Another way is to grasp quickly with stretched fingers and thumb (Fig. 1-9). The third way of grasping is to shape

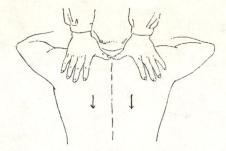

Fig. 1-6

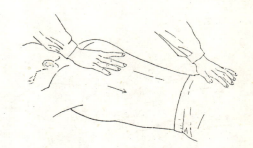

Fig. 1-7

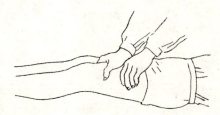

Fig. 1-8

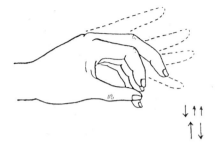

Fig. 1-9

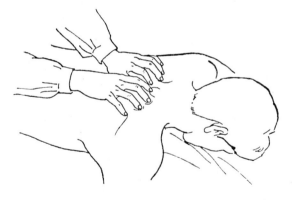

Fig. 1-10

the hand like a paw, grasp for a while, and then release (Fig. 1-10). This is often performed on the back and abdomen.

Category 2: Manipulations Smoothing the Meridians and Collaterals

1. Tapping

Tapping with the tip of the middle finger is usually done with strong force (Fig. 11). Tapping with the collected fingertips is usually done with low or medium intensity (Fig. 1-12).

Finger tapping is a basic manipulation, suitable for most acupoints to treat common diseases. The manipu-

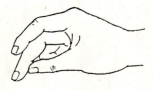

Fig. 1-11

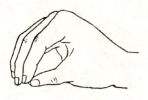

Fig. 1-12

lator should use the strength from the forearm and the wrist and tap at a speed of two to three times per second. Heavy taps should alternate with light taps, thus forming a rhythm. However, light taps should be fast, heavy taps a little slower. Rough manipulation should be avoided.

2. Digital Pressing

This is also a basic manipulation. Stretch the thumb, with the fingers open or crooked (the thumb resting on the index finger), press with tip of the thumb at an angle of 45° to 90° (Figs. 1-13, 14). Press in different directions.

3. Vibrating Manipulation

Finger vibration: The hand is in the same pose as that

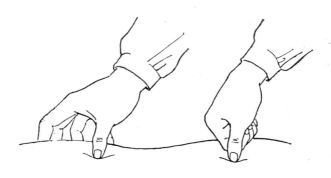

Fig. 1-13   Fig. 1-14

of finger tapping, but used for vibrating (Fig. 1-15). This is often used as a supplement to tapping or digital pressing.

Palm vibration (Fig. 1-16): This is usually used as a transient or connecting manipulation between two main manipulations.

4. Striking

Strike with cupped hand (Fig. 1-17) or half-clenched fist (Fig. 1-18) with varying force.

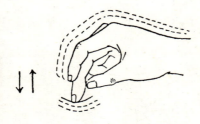

Fig. 1-15

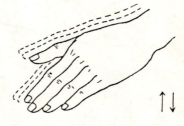

Fig. 1-16

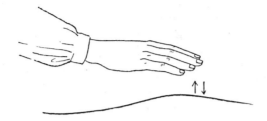

Fig. 1-17

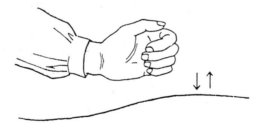

Fig. 1-18

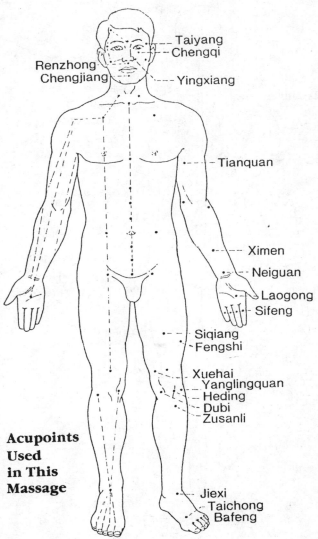

Acupoints Used in This Massage

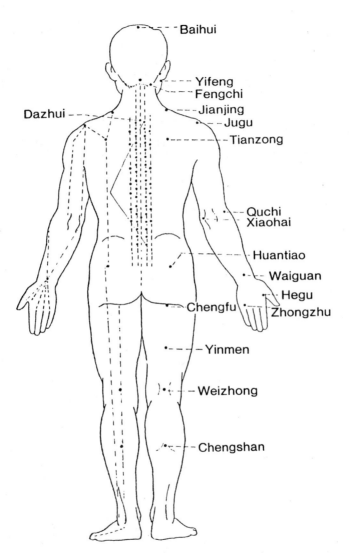

Massage Operation 1
Massage for Two People

Step 1.
The Sole: Stimulus-Input Regions

(Location) There are six stimulus-input regions on the sole, which are related to the heart, brain, liver, lung, spleen and kidney respectively (Fig. 2-1).

(Manipulation) The patient lies supine and relaxed. Push and squeeze the six regions with the thumb. (Stronger force should be applied to any area where lumps can be felt.) Begin with the kidney region and go on with the heart, brain, liver, lung, spleen regions, pushing and squeezing each region for 100 times or so.

(Indications) Kidney disease, diabetes, dyshormonism, hypertension, etc.

Note: The presence of lumps and a strong aching sensation while pressing in a certain region indicate abnormal corresponding organs and potential diseases. In that case, massage with stronger force.

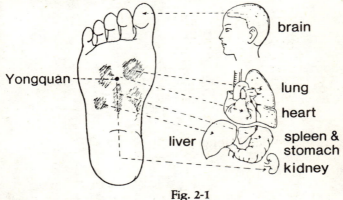

Fig. 2-1

Step 2.
Bafeng (EX-LE 10)

(Location) On the dorsum of the foot, in the depression on the webs between toes, proximal to the margin of the webs—eight points in all.

(Manipulation) Press and rub each point for one minute (Fig. 2-2).

(Indications) Swelling pain of the dorsum of the foot, peripheral neuritis, irregular menstruation.

(Transient Manipulation) Push and squeeze from the first of Bafeng (EX-LE 10) points to Taichong (LR 3) (see next step).

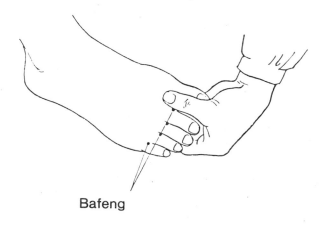

Bafeng

Fig. 2-2

Step 3.
Taichong (LR 3)

(Location) On the dorsum of the foot, in the depression distal to the junction of the first and second metatarsal bones.
(Manipulation) Press with the thumb (Fig. 2-3).
(Indications) Headaches, vertigo, hypertension, disorder of the liver-*qi*, irregular menstruation, uterine bleeding, mastitis.
(Transient Manipulation) Rub the dorsum of the foot with the palm until a burning heat sensation occurs.

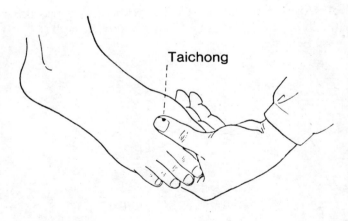

Fig. 2-3

Step 4.
Jiexi (ST 41)

(Location) On the dorsum of the foot, at the midpoint of the transverse crease of the ankle joint, in the depression between the tendons of the long extensor muscle of the toes and the long extensor muscle of the great toe, approximately at the level of the tip of the external malleolus.

(Manipulation) Press with the thumb (Fig. 2-4). The patient should feel a swelling ache spreading through the ankle joint and the dorsum of the foot.

(Indications) Headaches, myasthenia of the lower limbs, rheumarthritis.

(Transient Manipulation) Strike with hollow fist along the long extensor muscle of great toe to Zusanli (ST 36) (see next step).

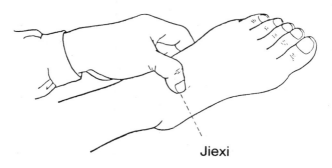

Fig. 2-4

Step 5.
Zusanli (ST 36)

(Location) When the knee is flexed, there is a depression lateral to the patellar ligament; three *cun* under this is Zusanli (ST 36).

(Manipulation) Press, press and move repeatedly; tap with fist (Fig. 2-5). The patient should feel an aching and light tingling sensation reaching the toe tips.

(Indications) Paralysis of the lower limbs, abdominal pain.

(Transient Manipulation) Strike with hollow fist downward from Zusanli (ST 36) to the ankle joint repeatedly for more than 10 times.

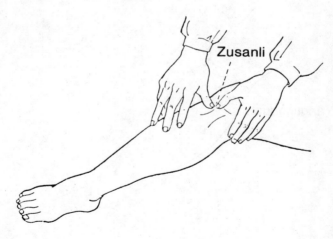

Fig. 2-5

Step 6.
Yanglingquan (GB 34)

(Location) In the depression anterior and inferior to the head of the fibula.

(Manipulation) Press and move repeatedly (Fig. 2-6). Aching sensation and light tingling will spread from the side of the leg to the dorsum of the foot.

(Indications) Pain in the knee joint, paralysis of the lower limbs.

(Transient Manipulation) Repeat grasping the side of the leg more than 10 times (Fig. 2-7).

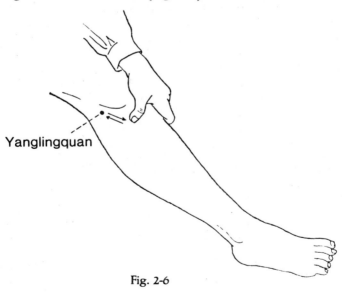

Fig. 2-6

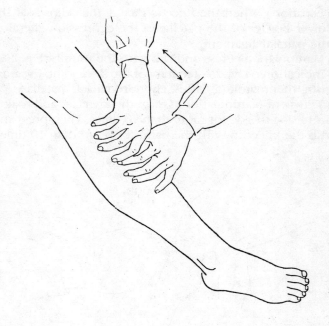

Fig. 2-7

Step 7.
Dubi (ST 35)

(Location) When the knee is flexed, the point is at the lower border of the patella, in the depression lateral to the patellar ligament.

(Manipulation) Press and rub with the thumb (Fig. 2-8).

(Indications) Hyperosteogeny of the knee joint, rheumatism, rheumatoid arthritis, chondromalacia patellae.

(Transient Manipulation) Grasp the kneecap and rock it from side to side for more than 10 times. Then press and rub the kneecap with the palm for more than 10 times.

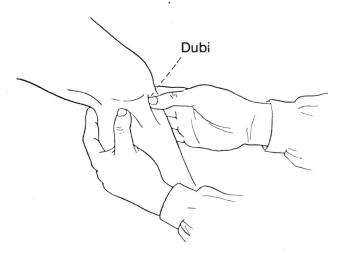

Fig. 2-8

Step 8.
Heding (EX-LE 2)

(Location) In the depression at the midpoint of the superior patellar border, as the knee is flexed.
(Manipulation) Press and move repeatedly (Fig. 2-9).
(Indications) Paralysis, knee joint disease, myasthenia of the lower limbs.

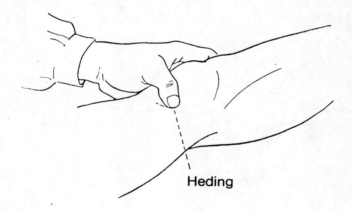

Fig. 2-9

Step 9.
Xuehai (SP 10)

(Location) When the knee is flexed, the point is two *cun* above the mediosuperior border of the patella.
(Manipulation) Rub the point with the palm clockwise and then counterclockwise for more than 10 times (Fig. 2-10).
(Indications) Anemia, irregular menstruation, dysfunctional uterine bleeding, dysmenorrhea.

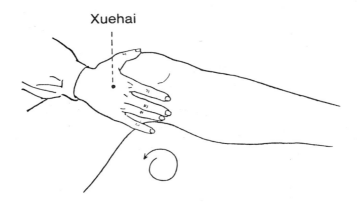

Fig. 2-10

Step 10.
Siqiang (EXTRA)

(Location) The point is 4.5 *cun* above the mediosuperior border of the patella.
(Manipulation) Rub with the thumb (Fig. 2-11).
(Indications) Myasthenia of the lower limbs, apoplectic hemiplegia.
(Transient Manipulation) Grasp the muscle on the two sides of the thigh from top downward for more than 10 times. Tap the anterior of the thigh from top downward with hollow fist for more than 10 times.

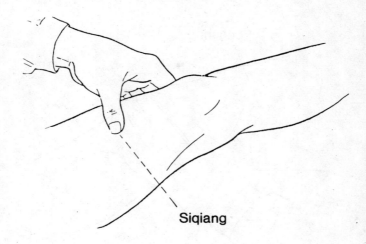

Fig. 2-11

Step 11.
Fengshi (GB 31)

(Location) When the patient is standing erect with the arms close to the sides, the point is where the tip of the middle finger touches.
(Manipulation) Press with the thumb with gradually increasing force (Fig. 2-12).
(Indications) Paralysis of the lower limbs, lumbago and pain in the leg, myasthenia.
(Transient Manipulation) Grasp muscles of the whole leg downward for several times.

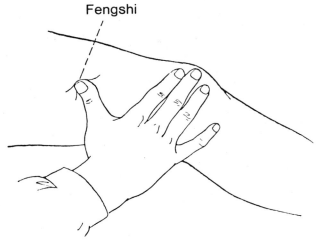

Fig. 2-12

Step 12.
The Pulsation Point of Femoral Artery

(Location) Below the inguinal ligament, where the pulse is felt.

(Manipulation) Press the two points with the two thumbs with gradually increasing force for one minute (Fig. 2-13). Keep the thumbs planted there until numbness spreads to the big toes.

(Indications) Angitis, rheumatic and rheumatoid arthritis, apoplectic paralysis, stasis of blood flow. This procedure is mainly meant to invigorate the circulation of blood and *qi*.

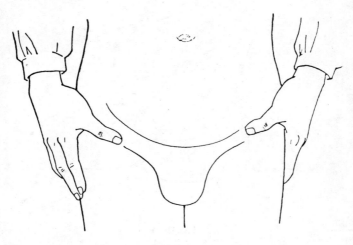

Fig. 2-13

(Transient Manipulation) Grab the patient's knee, fold the leg so that the heel touches the buttock and the knee is near the chest. Rock the knee from side to side (Fig. 2-14). Do this to the other leg. Then, grip one ankle with one hand, grip the knee of the same leg with the other hand and rock the leg from side to side and back and forth for more than 10 times (Fig. 2-15). After that, pull the leg several times. Do the same to the other leg and go on to next step.

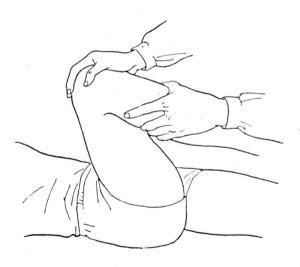

Fig. 2-14

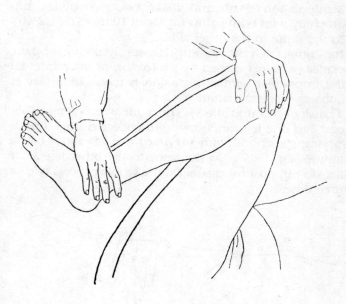

Fig. 2-15

Step 13.
Hip-Pushing

(Location) The sides of the hip.
(Manipulation) Push and shake one side of the hip forcefully with both palms for about 10 times (Fig. 2-16). Do the same to the other side.
(Indications) Gynecological diseases, lumbosacral pain, sciatica, scelalgia caused by protrusion of intervertebral disc, impotence, seminal emission, paralysis of the lower limbs, apoplectic hemiplegia.
(Transient Manipulation) The patient crooks his/her legs. Tap one leg randomly with collected fingertips at varying speed and with varying force for about half a minute (Fig. 2-17). Do the same to the other leg. After this, do hip-pushing again. Do the whole process two or three times.

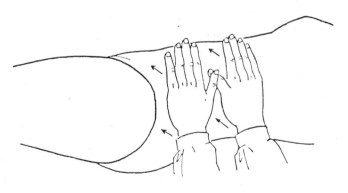

Fig. 2-16

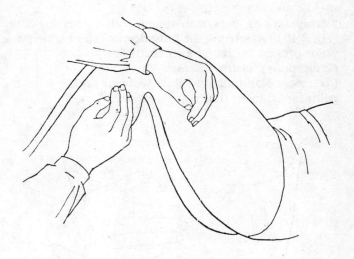

Fig. 2-17

Step 14.
Weiwan Region

(Location) Weiwan is the region between the xiphoid process and umbilicus, which is subdivided into upper, middle and lower parts.

(Manipulation) Press with finger with increasing force (Fig. 2-18). On sensing the pulsation of arteries, keep the point pressed for half a minute.

(Indications) Gastric diseases.

(Transient Manipulation) Rub Weiwan region with the palm for 20 to 30 times.

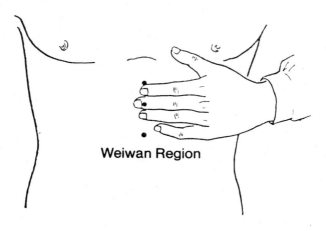

Fig. 2-18

Step 15.
Shangwan (RN 13)

(Location) On the midline of the abdomen, 5 *cun* above the umbilicus.
(Manipulation) Press and rub with the finger clockwise (Fig. 2-19).
(Indications) Acute and chronic gastritis, gastric dilatation, spasm of cardia of stomach.

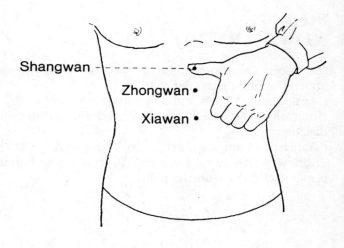

Fig. 2-19

Step 16.
Zhongwan (RN 12)

(Location) On the midline of the abdomen, 4 *cun* above the umbilicus (Fig. 2-19).
(Manipulation) Press and rub with the finger.
(Indications) Gastralgia, vomiting, hiccups, abdominal distension, diarrhea, gastritis, gastric ulcer, gastroptosis, acute gastric obstruction, dyspepsia.

Step 17.
Xiawan (RN 10)

(Location) On the midline of the abdomen, two *cun* above the umbilicus (Fig. 2-19).
(Manipulation) Press and rub with the finger.
(Indications) Gastralgia, vomiting, abdominal distension, dysentery.
(Transient Manipulation) Press Shangwan (RN 13), Zhongwan (RN 12), Xiawan (RN 10) repeatedly. Rub the upper abdomen with the palm.

Step 18.
Qihai (RN 6)

(Location) On the midline of the abdomen, 1.5 *cun* below the umbilicus (Fig. 2-20).

(Manipulation) Press with both thumbs simultaneously (the force should be light and heavy in turn) and repeatedly. Push the point with the thumbs toward left and right respectively. The patient will feel a swelling ache spreading to the upper and lower abdomen and the lumbus.

(Indications) Seminal emission, impotence, dysmenorrhea, irregular menstruation, abdominal distension, diarrhea, enuresis, frequency of micturition, retention of the urine, prostatitis.

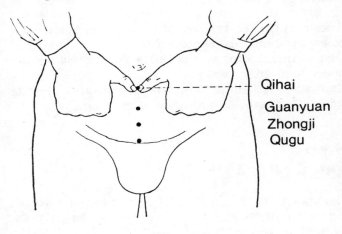

Fig. 2-20

Step 19.
Guanyuan (RN 4)

(Location) On the midline of the abdomen, three *cun* below the umbilicus (Fig. 2-20).
(Manipulation) Same as with step 18. The patient will feel a swelling ache spreading to the lower abdomen and pudendum.
(Indications) Irregular menstruation, dysmenorrhea, impotence, enuresis, abdominal pain, prolapse of the uterus, pruritus vulvae.

Step 20.
Zhongji (RN 3)

(Location) On the midline of the abdomen, four *cun* below the umbilicus (Fig. 2-20).
(Manipulation) Same as step 18. The patient will feel the pudendum getting heavy.
(Indications) Urethral obstruction, gonorrhea, female sterility, leukorrhagia, prolapase of the uterus.

Step 21.
Qugu (RN 2)

(Location) On the midline of the abdomen, five *cun* below the umbilicus, on the upper border of pubic symphysis (Fig. 2-20).
(Manipulation) Same as step 18. A swelling ache will

spread to the pudendum and anus.
(Indications) Impotence, morbid leukorrhea, anuresis.
(Transient Manipulation) Rub lower abdomen clockwise with the palm several times.

Step 22.
Daheng (SP 15)

(Location) Four *cun* lateral to the center of umbilicus.
(Manipulation) Press the two points with the thumbs for half a minute (Fig. 2-21). Push and rub them.
(Indications) Abdominal distension, diarrhea, constipation.
(Transient Manipulation) Rub both thumbs through the region from Shangwan (RN 13) to Qugu (RN 2) for

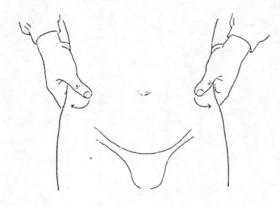

Fig. 2-21

more than 10 times (Fig. 2-22), then rub with the palm for 10 to 20 times (Fig. 2-23). Push the abdomen with stretched fingers for 10 to 20 times (Fig. 2-24). Rub the chest and abdomen for 10 to 20 times (Fig. 2-25).

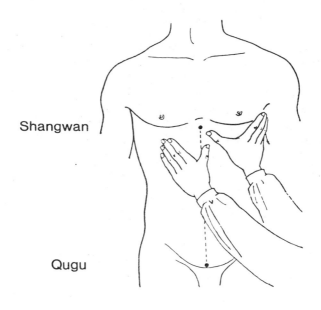

Fig. 2-22

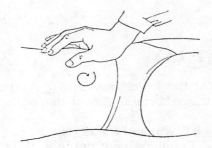

Fig. 2-23

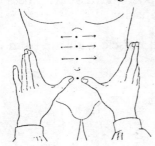

Fig. 2-24

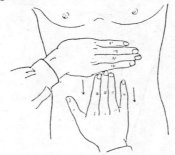

Fig. 2-25

Step 23.
Qihu (ST 13)

(Location) At the lower border of the middle of the clavicle, four *cun* lateral to the midline of the chest and abdomen.

(Manipulation) Press and knead (Fig. 2-26).

(Indications) Coughing with dyspnea, chest pain, fullness in the chest and hypochondrium, weakness of the heart, decrease of vital capacity.

(Transient Manipulation)

1. Knead greater pectoral muscle with the palm for 10 to 20 times (Fig. 2-27).

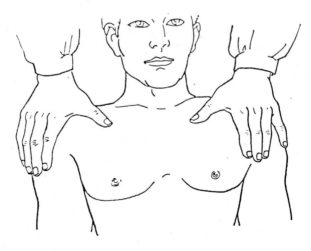

Fig. 2-26

2. Push with the thumbs along the costal foveas on both sides. Perform this for 3 to 4 times (Fig. 2-28).
3. Rub the chest with the palm for 3 to 5 times (Fig. 2-29).
4. Cup the hand and clap it on the chest for 10 to 20 times (Fig. 2-30).

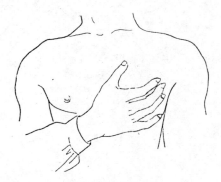

Fig. 2-27

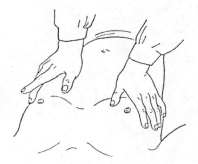

Fig. 2-28

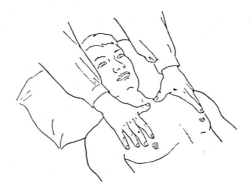

Fig. 2-29

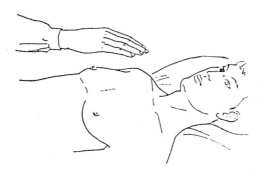

Fig. 2-30

52

Step 24.
Danzhong (RN 17)

(Location) On the anterior midline, midway between the nipples.
(Manipulation) Tap with collected fingertips (Fig. 2-31).
(Indications) Chest pain, chest distress, deficiency of milk secretion, intercostal neuralgia, angina pectoris, coughing, asthma, hiccups, mastitis. Also excites facial muscles and prevents hyperplasia of mammary glands.

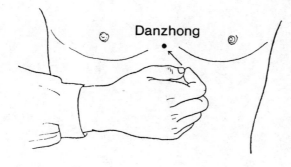

Fig. 2-31

Step 25.
Tiantu (RN 22)

(Location) In the center of the suprasternal fossa.
(Manipulation) Press with the thumb (Fig. 2-32).
(Indications) Bronchial asthma, bronchitis, laryngopharyngitis, thyroid enlargement, spasm of diaphragm, disease of esophagus, neurogenic vomiting, disease of vocal cord.
Note: The above massage methods on the chest, if practiced persistently, can prevent diseases of the lung and esophagus.
(Transient Manipulation) Grasp muscles on the arm from top downward to the hand.

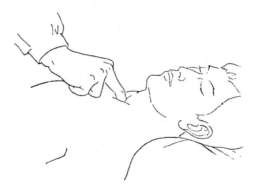

Fig. 2-32

Step 26.
Hegu (LI 4)

(Location) On the dorsum of the hand, between the first and second metacarpal bones, approximately in the middle of the second metacarpal bone on the radial side.
(Manipulation) Press with finger, together with Quchi (LI 11) point (see step 33). (Fig. 2-33)
(Indications) Common cold, facial paralysis, hemiplegia, neurasthenia, tonsillitis, facial paralysis, toothaches, abdominal pain, palsy of hand and various pain. Also prevents hypertension.

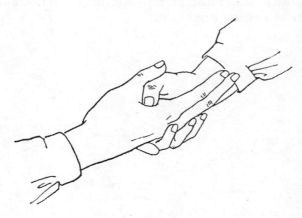

Fig. 2-33

Step 27.
Zhongzhu (KI 15)

(Location) When the fist is clenched, the point is on the dorsum of the hand between the fourth and fifth metacarpal bones, in the depression proximal to the metacarpophalangeal joint.

(Manipulation) Press and rub with the thumb (Fig. 2-34).

(Indications) Hypertension, coronary heart disease, apoplexy.

Note: Zhongzhu (KI 15) is an important point for reducing blood pressure.

(Transient Manipulation) Rub dorsum of the hand until there is a burning sensation.

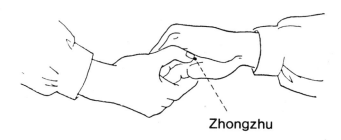

Fig. 2-34

Step 28.
Sifeng (EX-UE 10)

(Location) On the palmar surface, in the midpoint of the transverse creases of the proximal interphalangeal joints of the index, middle, ring and little fingers—eight points in all on the two hands.

(Manipulation) Hold the point between a finger and the thumb and pull (Fig. 2-35).

(Indications) Pertussis, malnutrition and indigestion in children, digital arthritis, apoplexy, hypertension.

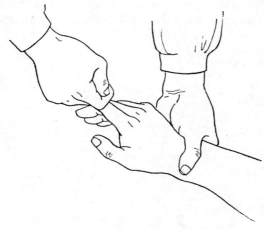

Fig. 2-35

Step 29.
Laogong (PC 8)

(Location) On the transverse crease of the palm. When the fist is clenched, the point is just below the tip of the middle finger.

(Manipulation) Knead with the thumb (Fig. 2-36).

(Indications) Psychosis, epilepsy, insomnia, heatstroke, vomiting, stomatitis, hypertension, coronary heart disease.

(Transient Manipulation) Hold the patient's wrist with both hands, pull and turn it in different directions (Fig. 2-37). Do this for more than 10 times. Press Ximen (PC 4) (see step 32) with the thumb for several times.

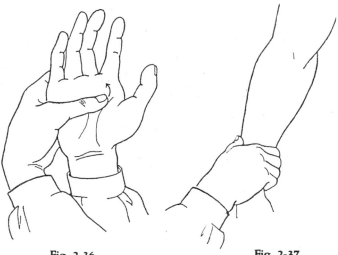

Fig. 2-36   Fig. 2-37

Step 30.
Neiguan (PC 6)

(Location) Two *cun* above the transverse crease of the wrist, between the tendons of the long palmar muscle and radial flexor muscle.

(Manipulation) Press and rub with the thumb (Fig. 2-38). A swelling ache should spread to the upper arm.

(Indications) Pain in chest and hypochondrium, stomachache, shock, nausea, sore throat, hysteria, arrhythmia, hypertension, apoplexy.

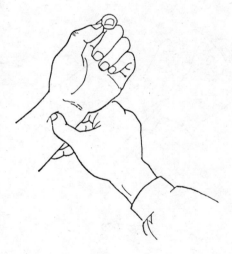

Fig. 2-38

Step 31.
Waiguan (SJ 5)

(Location) Two *cun* above the transverse crease of the dorsum of wrist, between the radius and ulna.
(Manipulation) Press and rub with the thumb (Fig. 2-39). A swelling ache should spread to the upper arm.
(Indications) Common cold, pneumonia, deafness, migraine, hypertension, coronary heart disease. Also prevents apoplexy.

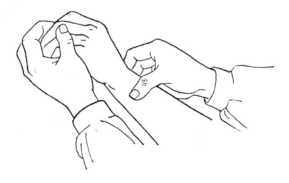

Fig. 2-39

Step 32.
Ximen (PC 4)

(Location) Five *cun* above the transverse crease of the wrist between the tendons of the long palmar muscle and radial flexor muscle.

(Manipulation) Press and stroke with the thumb (Fig. 2-40).

(Indications) Angina pectoris, tachycardia, pleurisy, mastitis, hypertension, apoplectic paralysis.

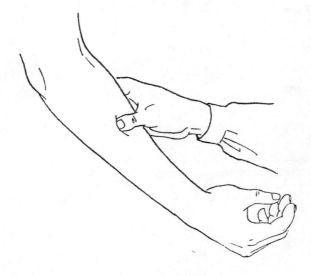

Fig. 2-40

Step 33.
Quchi (LI 11)

(Location) When the elbow is flexed, the point is in the depression at the lateral end of the transverse cubital crease.

(Manipulation) Press and stroke (Fig. 2-41).

(Indications) Apoplectic hemiplegia, arthralgia of the limbs, hypertension, pyrexia, measles, lumbago and back pain.

(Transient Manipulation) Grasp the anterior part of the arm, stroke borders of muscles with the thumb (Fig. 2-42).

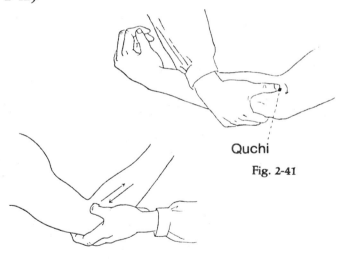

Quchi

Fig. 2-41

Fig. 2-42

Step 34.
Xiaohai (SI 8)

(Location) When the elbow is flexed, the point is located in the depression between the olecranon of the ulna and the medial epicondyle of the humerus.

(Manipulation) Stroke with the four fingers, not using the thumb (Fig. 2-43).

(Indications) Hypertension, heart disease, apoplexy, brachial palsy, arthralgia of neck, shoulder and elbow. Also does much to prevent apoplexy.

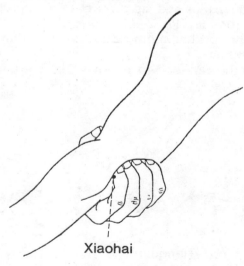

Fig. 2-43

Step 35.
Tianquan (PC 2)

(Location) Two *cun* below the level of the anterior axillary fold, between the two heads of the biceps muscle of the arm.
(Manipulation) Press and stroke (Fig. 2-44).
(Indications) Hypertension, brachial palsy, apoplexy, heart disease, coughing.
(Transient Manipulation)
1. Scrub for 5 to 10 times (Fig. 2-45).
2. Cup the hands and tap the arm from opposite sides for 5 to 10 times (Fig. 2-46).
3. Roll the hand along the arm for 5 to 10 times (Fig. 2-47).
4. Grasp the arm for 5 to 10 times (Fig. 2-48).

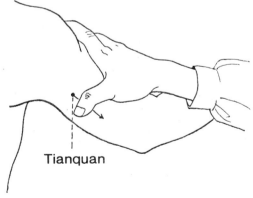

Fig. 2-44

5. Holding the patient's arm under the armpit, take the patient's shoulder with both hands, knead it forcefully (Fig. 2-49). Knead and shake it for 10 to 20 times.

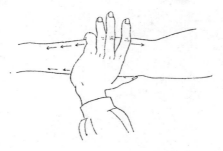

Fig. 2-45

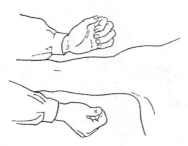

Fig. 2-46

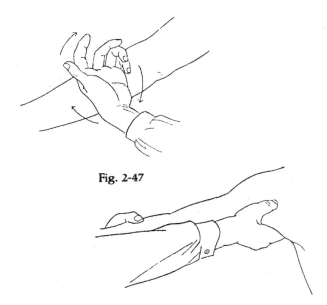

Fig. 2-47

Fig. 2-48

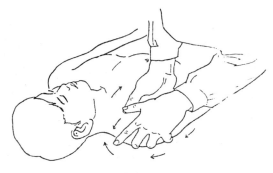

Fig. 2-49

Step 36.
Carotid

(Location) The point is 0.5 *cun* above the clavicle, one third of the length of the clavicle from its medial end, where the pulse is felt.

(Manipulation) Press each of the two points with a thumb with increasing force for half a minute (Fig. 2-50). The patient should feel a swelling ache and tingling spreading to the arms and back, and feel a heat stream flow to the head when the thumbs are released.

(Indications) Hypertension, cerebral ischemia, heart disease, apoplexy, brachial palsy.

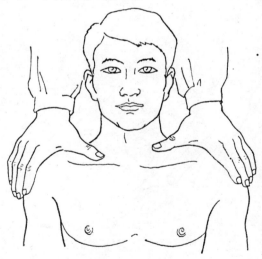

Fig. 2-50

Step 37.
Taiyang (EX-HN 5)

(Location) In the depression about one *cun* posterior to the midpoint between the lateral end of the eyebrow and the outer canthus.

(Manipulation) Press it together with Cuanzhu (BL 2) (at the medial end of the eyebrow at the supraorbital notch) and the anterior hairline with the fingers (Fig. 2-51).

(Indications) Headaches, trigeminal neuralgia, common cold, facial paralysis, hypertension.

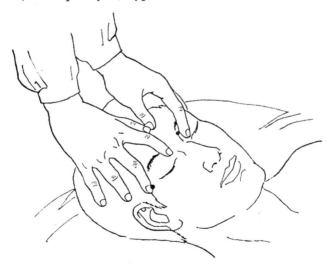

Fig. 2-51

Step 38.
Yingxiang (LI 20)

(Location) In the nasolabial groove, at the level of the midpoint of the lateral border of ala nasi.

(Manipulation) Press for half a minute, rub it for 10 to 20 times. Then from there, stroke across the face for 10 to 20 times. (Fig. 2-52)

(Indications) Nasal diseases, facial paralysis, trigeminal neuralgia, facial spasm.

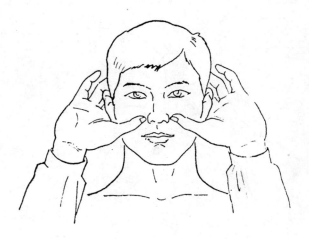

Fig. 2-52

Step 39.
Chengqi (ST 1)

(Location) With the eyes looking straight forward, the point is directly below the pupil, between the eyeball and the infraorbital ridge.
(Manipulation) Press with a vibrating finger (Fig. 2-53).
(Indications) Myopia, blepharospasm, optic atrophy, trigeminal neuralgia, facial hemiparalysis.
(Transient Manipulation) Knead the face with both palms for more than 10 times.

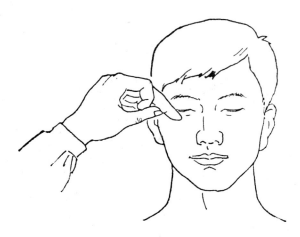

Fig. 2-53

Step 40.
Chengjiang (RN 24)

(Location) In the depression at the midpoint of the mentolabial groove.
(Manipulation) Press with a vibrating index finger (Fig. 2-54).
(Indications) Trigeminal neuralgia, facial paralysis, hypertension.

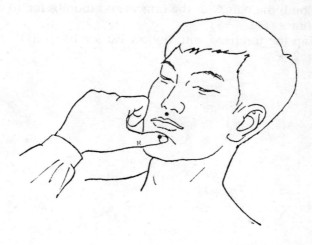

Fig. 2-54

Step 41.
Renzhong (DU 26)

(Location) A little above the midpoint of the philtrum, near the nostrils (Fig. 2-54).

(Manipulation) Press with a vibrating index finger.

(Indications) Hypertension, shock, coma, psychosis, epilepsy, heatstroke, suffocation, respiratory failure, coronary heart disease. This is an important acupoint for first aid.

(Transient Manipulation)

1. Comb the hair with the fingers and thumbs for 10 to 20 times (Fig. 2-55).

2. Tap the forehead with hollow fist for 10 to 20 times (Fig. 2-56).

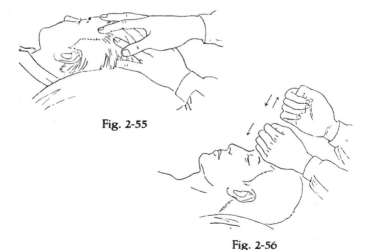

Fig. 2-55

Fig. 2-56

Step 42.
Yintang (EX-HN 3)

(Location) Midway between the medial ends of the two eyebrows.
(Manipulation) Rub with both thumbs (Fig. 2-57).
(Indications) Headaches, insomnia, vertigo, nasal disease, common cold, hypertension.
(Transient Manipulation) Continue to rub the area from Yintang (EX-HN 3) to anterior hairline. Press the hairline with fingertips and gradually move to Touwei (ST 8) (see next step).

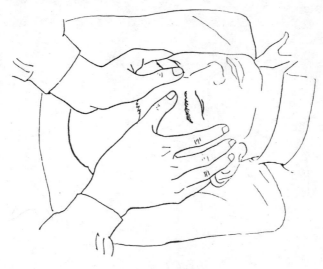

Fig. 2-57

Step 43.
Touwei (ST 8)

(Location) The point is 0.5 *cun* within the anterior hairline at the corner of the forehead.
(Manipulation) Press with the thumb (Fig. 2-58).
(Indications) Headaches, cerebral anoxia, vertigo, hypertension.
(Transient Manipulation) Pinch the eyebrow area with the thumb and index finger from the medial end to the side for several times (Fig. 2-59).

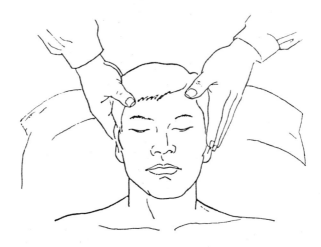

Fig. 2-58

Step 44.
Sizhukong (SJ 23)

(Location) In the depression at the lateral end of the eyebrow (Fig. 2-59).
(Manipulation) Press with the thumb.
(Indications) Hypertension, apoplexy, facial paralysis, strabismus, influenza, headaches.
(Transient Manipulation) Rub from Sizhukong (SJ 23) to Taiyang (EX-HN 5). Rub Taiyang (EX-HN 5) for 10 to 20 times. Rub from Taiyang (EX-HN 5) to Yifeng (SJ 17) (see next step).

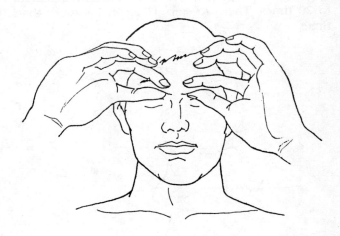

Fig. 2-59

Step 45.
Yifeng (SJ 17)

(Location) Posterior to the earlobe, in the depression between the mandible and mastoid process.

(Manipulation) Press and rub with index finger (Fig. 2-60).

(Indications) Tinnitus, deafness, facial paralysis, parotitis, mandibular arthritis, toothaches, hypertension, eye diseases.

(Transient Manipulation) Rub each cheek with a palm for 10 to 20 times. Tap randomly at the face with fingertips. Rub the face with the palm and fingers for 10 to 20 times. Then do step 41 again for more than 10 times.

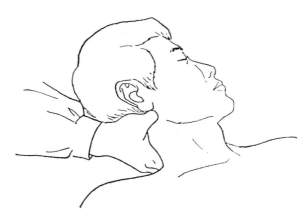

Fig. 2-60

Step 46.
Qianding (DU 21)

(Location) On the middle line of the head, 1.5 *cun* anterior to the midpoint of the line connecting the apexes of the two auricles.
(Manipulation) Press with the finger (Fig. 2-61).
(Indications) Apoplexy, hypertension.
(Transient Manipulation) Press the area between Qianding (DU 21) and Baihui (DU 20) (see next step).

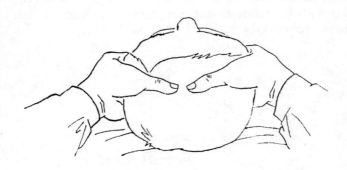

Fig. 2-61

Step 47.
Baihui (DU 20)

(Location) On the middle line of the head, approximately on the midpoint of the line connecting the apexes of the two auricles.

(Manipulation) Press with the thumb (Fig. 2-61).

(Indications) Hypertension, apoplexy, coma, headaches, vertigo, psychosis, prolapse of the uterus, prolapse of the anus, paralysis, myasthenia.

(Transient Manipulation) Push with thumb from anterior hairline to Baihui (DU 20) for 10 to 20 times. Squeeze the part of scalp from anterior hairline to Baihui (DU 20) with two thumbs for 5 to 10 times. Then rub the three areas on the scalp as Fig. 2-62 shows.

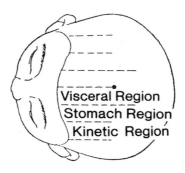

Fig. 2-62

Step 48.
The Ear

(Manipulation) Hold the auricle between the thumb and the fingers and rub it for 30 to 50 times. Then rub the antilobium, earlobe, antitragus in the same way for 10 to 20 times. The rubbing should gain speed gradually until the patient feels feverish over the body, in order to give enough stimulation to the acupoints on the ear which correspond to various organs (Fig. 2-63).

(Transient Manipulation) Seal the antrum auris with index finger for half a minute and put out the finger suddenly. Tap the forehead with hollow fists for 30 to

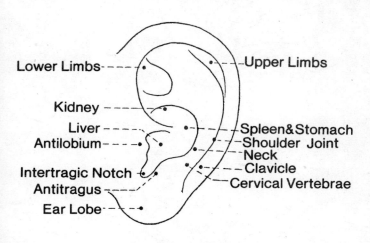

Fig. 2-63

50 times (Fig. 2-64). Comb the hair with the thumbs and fingers. With stretched fingers and thumbs, grasp the scalp and forehead bouncingly and speedily for more than 10 times (Fig. 2-65).

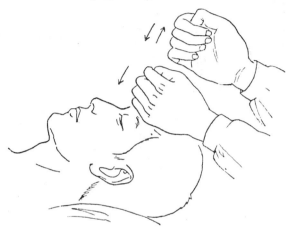

Fig. 2-64

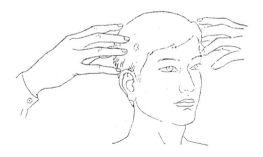

Fig. 2-65

Step 49.
Fengchi (GB 20)

(Location) In the depression between the upper ends of sternocleidomastoid and trapezius muscles, 0.5 *cun* within the hairline.

(Manipulation) With the patient sitting up, press the point with finger (Fig. 2-66).

(Indications) Common cold, headaches, vertigo, stiffness and pain of nape, eye diseases, rhinitis, tinnitus, deafness, hypertension, epilepsy, hemiplegia, encephalopathy.

(Transient Manipulation) Rub Fengchi (GB 20).

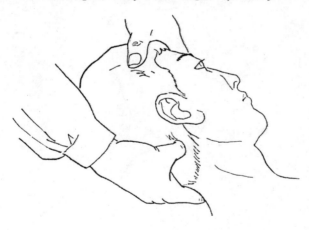

Fig. 2-66

Step 50.
Fengfu (DU 16)

(Location) One *cun* directly above the midpoint of the posterior hairline, directly below the external occipital protuberance, in the depression between the trapezius muscle of both sides.

(Manipulation) Press and rub with the finger (Fig. 2-67).

(Indications) Psychosis, insomnia, sequelae of apoplexy.

(Transient Manipulation) Knead the area between Fengfu (DU 16) and Dazhui (DU 14) (see next step), moving from Fengfu (DU 16) downward. Knead the left and right sides of the neck.

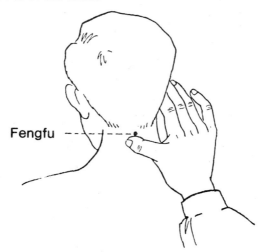

Fig. 2-67

Step 51.
Dazhui (DU 14)

(Location) Below the spinous process of the seventh cervical vertebra, approximately at the level of the shoulders.

(Manipulation) Press with the thumb (Fig. 2-68).

(Indications) Common cold, fever, coughing, asthma, stiffness of nape, stiffness of back, manic-depressive psychosis, general myasthenia.

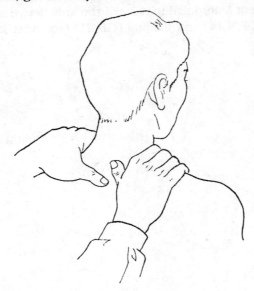

Fig. 2-68

Step 52.
Yiming (EX-HN 14)

(Location) One *cun* posterior to Yifeng (SJ 17) (see step 45).

(Manipulation) Tap with collected fingertips (Fig. 2-69). The patient will feel a pulsation spreading to the foot when tapped.

(Indications) Hypertension, optic atrophy, tinnitus, vertigo, insomnia.

(Transient Manipulation) Knead the area between Yiming (EX-HN 14) and Jianjing (GB 21) (see next step).

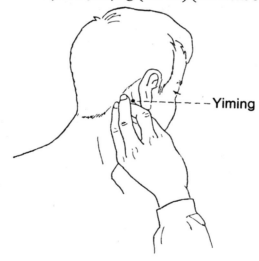

Fig. 2-69

Step 53.
Jianjing (GB 21)

(Location) Midway between Dazhui (DU 14) (see step 51) and the acromion, in the depression of the trapezeus.
(Manipulation) Press heavily with the thumb (Fig. 2-70).
(Indications) Diseases of the shoulder and back, mastitis.
(Transient Manipulation) Grasp the shoulder for 20 to 30 times. Grasp the area around Jianjing (GB 21) and lift it (Fig. 2-71).

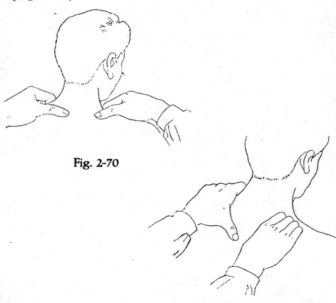

Fig. 2-70

Fig. 2-71

Step 54.
Jugu (LI 16)

(Location) In the upper aspect of the shoulder, in the depression between the acromial extremity of the clavicle and the scapular spine.

(Manipulation) Press and rub with the thumb (Fig. 2-72).

(Indications) Cervical spondylopathy, scapulohumeral periarthritis, disease of soft tissue, hematemesis, lymphoid tuberculosis, pain in the arm, apoplectic paralysis, hypertension, excessive sweating.

(Transient Manipulation) Rub from Jugu (LI 16) to Tianzong (SI 11) (see next step).

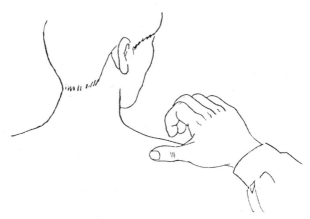

Fig. 2-72

Step 55.
Tianzong (SI 11)

(Location) In the infrascapular fossa, at the junction of the upper and middle third of the distance between the lower border of the scapular spine and the inferior angle of the scapula.
(Manipulation) Press and rub with the thumb (Fig. 2-73).
(Indications) Apoplectic paralysis, cervical spondylopathy, scapulohumeral periarthritis, asthma, brachial palsy.
(Transient Manipulation) Press the scapulae and the thoracic vertebrae from top downward for more than 10 times. Tap the acromions with hollow fist and cupped hand for 20 to 30 times.

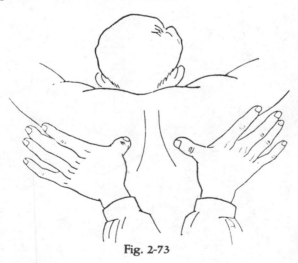

Fig. 2-73

Step 56.
The Back

(Manipulation) The patient lies prone. Roll the hand over the back for several times (Fig. 2-74). Rub the back with heel of the hand for 10 to 20 times (Fig. 2-75). Push Huatuojiaji (EX-B 2) points (see next step) downward with the thumb for 10 to 20 times (Fig. 2-76). Pinch the last two Huatuojiaji (EX-B 2) points with the thumbs and index fingers and push to the first two points (Fig. 2-77). Repeat 2 to 4 times. Pinch and pull up each Huatuojiaji (EX-B 2) point once.

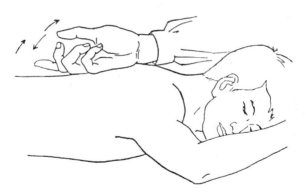

Fig. 2-74

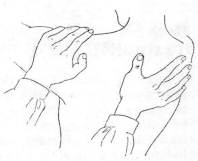

Fig. 2-75

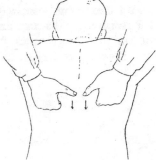

Fig. 2-76

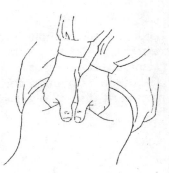

Fig. 2-77

Step 57.
Huatuojiaji (EX-B 2)

(Location) A group of 34 points on both sides of the spinal column, 0.5 *cun* lateral to the lower border of each spinous process from the first thoracic vertebra to the fifth lumbar vertebra.
(Manipulation) Pinch every point.
(Indications) Arthrosis of vertebrae, diseases of visceral organs such as stomachache and coughing. Points on the upper part are indicated for respiratory diseases and cardiovascular diseases, points on the middle part for digestive diseases, points on the lower part for diseases of the loin, abdomen and lower limb.

Step 58.
Feishu (BL 13)

(Location) The point is 1.5 *cun* lateral to the lower border of the spinous process of the third thoracic vertebra.
(Manipulation) Press and rub with the finger (Fig. 2-78).
(Indications) Common cold, coughing, asthma, pulmonary heart disease, night sweating and diseases of the back.

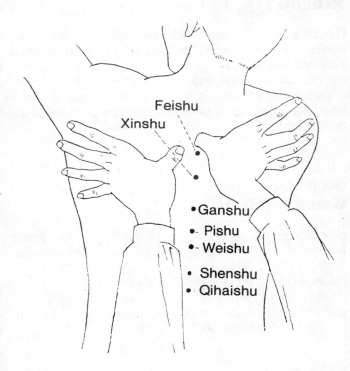

Fig. 2-78

Step 59.
Xinshu (BL 15)

(Location) The point is 1.5 *cun* lateral to the lower border of the spinous process of the fifth thoracic vertebra (Fig. 2-78).
(Manipulation) Press and rub with the finger.
(Indications) Palpitation due to fright, vexation, amnesia, coughing, angina pectoris, arrhythmia, tachycardia, neurasthenia.

Step 60.
Ganshu (BL 18)

(Location) The point is 1.5 *cun* lateral to the lower border of the spinous process of the ninth thoracic vertebra (Fig. 2-78).
(Manipulation) Press and rub with the finger.
(Indications) Diseases of the liver and gallbladder, hypochondriac pain, stomachache, hematemesis, pain in the vertebral column and backache.

Step 61.
Pishu (BL 20)

(Location) The point is 1.5 *cun* lateral to the lower border of the spinous process of the eleventh thoracic vertebra (Fig. 2-78).

(Manipulation) Press and rub with the finger.
(Indications) Abdominal distension, vomiting, dysentery, edema, weakness of the spleen and the stomach, indigestion, chronic diarrhea, hepatitis, backache, anemia.

Step 62.
Weishu (BL 21)

(Location) The point is 1.5 *cun* lateral to the lower border of the spinous process of the twelfth thoracic vertebra (Fig. 2-78).
(Manipulation) Press and rub with the finger.
(Indications) Pain in chest and hypochondrium, epigastralgia, abdominal distension, gastric disorder causing nausea, vomiting, borborygmi, weakness of the spleen and stomach, indigestion, chronic diarrhea.

Step 63.
Shenshu (BL 23)

(Location) The point is 1.5 *cun* lateral to the lower border of the spinous process of the second lumbar vertebra (Fig. 2-78).
(Manipulation) Press and rub with the finger.
(Indications) Urinary tract infection, impotence, seminal emission, irregular menstruation, morbid leukorrhea, retention of urine, weakness of kidney-*qi*, asthma, tinnitus, deafness, chronic diarrhea, chronic lumbago and back pain, cerebral ischemia, hypertension.

Step 64.
Qihaishu (BL 24)

(Location) The point is 1.5 *cun* lateral to the lower border of the spinous process of the third lumbar vertebra (Fig. 2-78).

(Manipulation) Press and rub with the finger.

(Indications) Abdominal pain, abdominal distension, borborygmi, diarrhea, constipation, lumbago, impotence, hypertension.

Note: The above six "shu" points are selected from the group of "shu" points of which each is located 1.5 *cun* lateral to the spinous process of each vertebra. Massage on all these "shu" points can be applied.

(Transient Manipulation)

1. Strike the back with hollow fist from top downward for 3 to 5 times (Fig. 2-79).

2. Strike the back with cupped hand from top downward for 3 to 5 times (Fig. 2-80).

3. Strike the back with the hand held perpendicularly like a cleaver from top downward for 3 to 5 times (Fig. 2-81).

4. Slap the back with the hand for 3 to 5 times (Fig. 2-82).

5. Grasp the back with the fingers and thumbs for 3 to 5 times (Fig. 2-83).

6. Push muscles on the back with the palm from top downward for 3 to 5 times (Fig. 2-84).

7. Scrub the back (Fig. 2-85).

8. Grasp muscles lateral to the vertebrae (Fig. 2-86).

This process enables all points on back to get some stimulation.

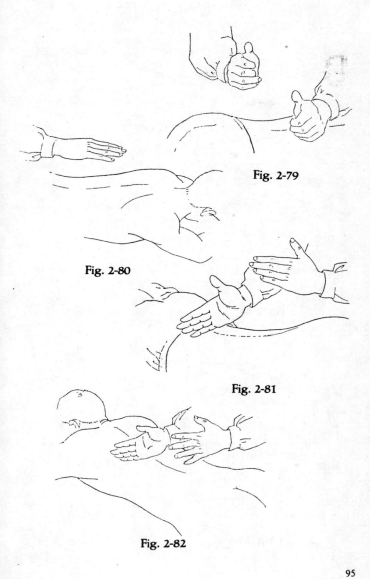

Fig. 2-79

Fig. 2-80

Fig. 2-81

Fig. 2-82

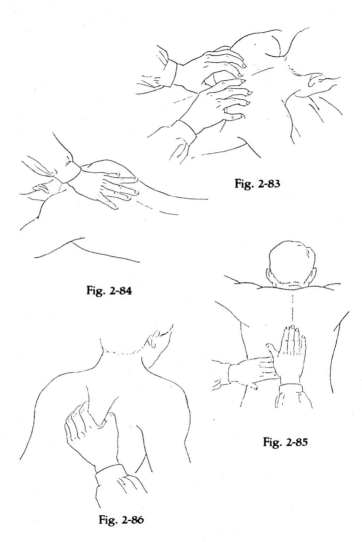

Fig. 2-83

Fig. 2-84

Fig. 2-85

Fig. 2-86

Step 65.
The Lumbus

(Manipulation) Press lumbar muscle with the thumb for half a minute. Push, rub, squeeze, and stroke with the two thumbs as if rowing a boat (the lumbar muscle being the boat, the thumbs the oars) for several times (Fig. 2-87).

(Transient Manipulation) Tap lumbosacral portion with hollow fist for 5 to 10 times.

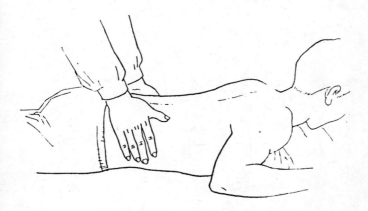

Fig. 2-87

Step 66.
Huantiao (GB 30)

(Location) At the junction of the lateral one third and medial two thirds of the distance between the great trochanter and the hiatus of the sacrum.

(Manipulation) Rub with the elbow (Fig. 2-88).

(Indications) Sciatica, lumbago and pain in the leg, paraparesis, paralysis, disease of the kidney.

(Transient Manipulation) Rub from Huantiao (GB 30) downward to the Achilles tendon for 5 to 10 times. Then press with finger along the same route.

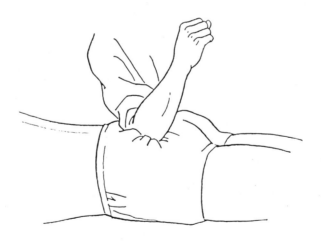

Fig. 2-88

Step 67.
Chengfu (BL 36)

(Location) In the middle of the inferior gluteal crease.
(Manipulation) Press and stroke with the finger (Fig. 2-89).
(Indications) Lumbosacral pain, sciatica, paralysis of the lower limbs, anuresis, constipation, apoplectic hemiplegia, myasthenia of the lower limbs, decreased renal function.
(Transient Manipulation) Press with finger along the route from Chengfu (BL 36) to Yinmen (BL 37) (see next step).

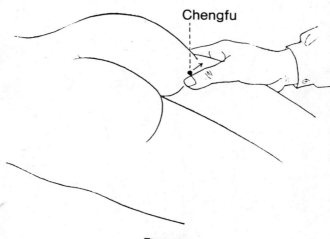

Fig. 2-89

Step 68.
Yinmen (BL 37)

(Location) Six *cun* below Chengfu (BL 36) on the line joining Chengfu (BL 36) and Weizhong (BL 40) (see next step).

(Manipulation) Press with the two thumbs simultaneously (Fig. 2-90).

(Indications) Lumbago and back pain, sciatica, paralysis of the lower limb.

(Transient Manipulation) Press from Yinmen (BL 37) to Weizhong (BL 40) (see next step).

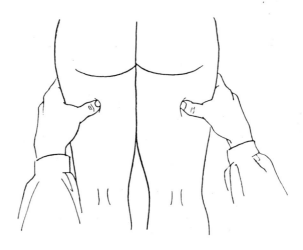

Fig. 2-90

Step 69.
Weizhong (BL 40)

(Location) Midpoint of the transverse crease of the popliteal fossa, between the tendons of the biceps muscle of the thigh and the semitendinous muscle.
(Manipulation) Press with the finger (Fig. 2-91).
(Indications) Seminal emission, impotence, urinary obstruction, acute and chronic lumbago, sciatica, diseases of the lower limbs and knee joints, hyperosteogeny of the knee joint, acute gastroenteritis, vomiting, diarrhea, abdominal pain, disease of the kidney.
(Transient Manipulation) Press from Weizhong (BL 40) to Chengshan (BL 57).

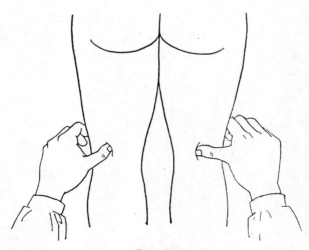

Fig. 2-91

Step 70.
Chengshan (BL 57)

(Location) Directly below the belly of gastrocnemius muscle, on the line joining Weizhong (BL 40) and Achilles tendon, about eight *cun* below Weizhong.

(Manipulation) Press with the thumb (Fig. 2-92).

(Indications) Lumbago and pain in the leg, sciatica, spasm of leg muscle, paralysis, hemorrhoids, prolapse of the anus.

(Transient Manipulation) Pinch Achilles tendon for 10 to 20 times (Fig. 2-93). Grasp muscles of the whole leg, repeating this from top downward for 10 to 20 times (Fig. 2-94).

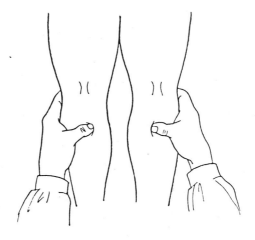

Fig. 2-92

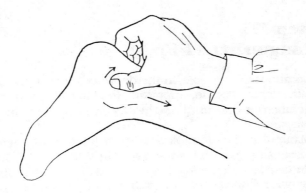

Fig. 2-93

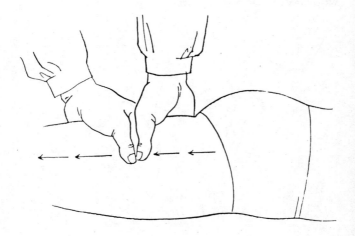

Fig. 2-94

Step 71.
Yongquan (KI 1)

(Location) On the sole, in the depression when the foot is in plantar flexion, approximately at the junction of the anterior one third and posterior two thirds of the sole.

(Manipulation) Rub rapidly with the palm until there is a feverish sensation on the sole (Fig. 2-95).

(Ending Manipulation) Tap the muscles on the whole leg with hollow fist for more than 10 times (with stronger force on acupoints). Knock with cupped hand in the same way for more than 10 times. Then rub the whole body for 5 to 10 times (Fig. 2-96).

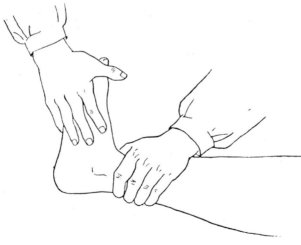

Fig. 2-95

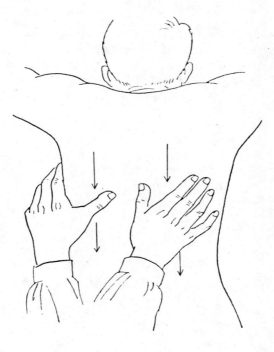

Fig. 2-96

Massage Operation 2
Self-Massage

Step 1.
Sitting, rub rapidly the sole of the left foot against the dorsum of the right foot for 20 to 30 times. Then rub rapidly the sole of the right foot against the dorsum of the left foot for 20 to 30 times (Fig. 3-1). A burning sensation will be felt.

These actions speed up blood circulation in the foot —the end of the body—and stimulate the six regions on the sole relating to six visceral organs. This can relieve or cure kidney disease, diabetes, hypertension, etc. It is also a good way to recover from tiredness.

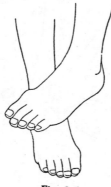

Fig. 3-1

Step 2.
Strike Zusanli (ST 36) of the right leg with the heel of the the left foot for 10 to 20 times; then strike Zusanli (ST 36) of the left leg with the heel of the right foot for 10 to 20 times (Fig. 3-2). This should be done with rather heavy force. This method is indicated in stomach diseases, insomnia, hypertension, and heart disease. This

method also exercises the hip joint, preventing senile aseptic necrosis of the head of the femur, reducing the chance of breaking the femur and tibia for old people.

Step 3.
Rub Zusanli (ST 36) and anterior tibial muscle of the right leg with Achilles tendon of the left leg for 10 to 20 times (Fig. 3-3). Do the same to the left leg for 10 to 20 times. This method is indicated in stomach diseases and hypertension. It also exercises the knee joint and hip joint and prevents the troubles of the joints.

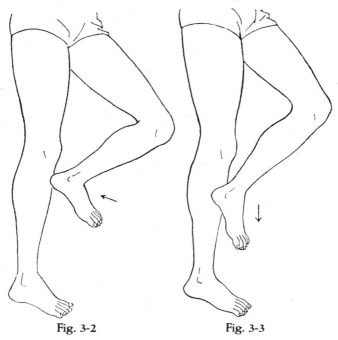

Fig. 3-2   Fig. 3-3

Step 4.
Pinch and rub Dubi (ST 35) with the thumb and index finger for 10 to 20 times (Fig. 3-4). Indications: inflammation of the knee joint, hyperosteogeny of the knee joint. Also prevents apoplectic hemiplegia.

Step 5.
Knead the kneecap with the palm clockwise for 10 to 20 times and counterclockwise for 10 to 20 times (Fig. 3-5). Indications: inflammation of the knee joint, hyperosteogeny of the knee joint. Also prevents chondromalacia patellae, gonarthrosis.

Step 6.
Grasp the calf from top downward and from bottom upward repeatedly for 10 to 20 times (Fig. 3-6). Indication: posterior crural spasm.

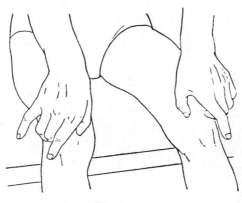

Fig. 3-4

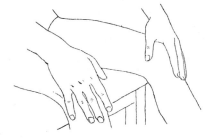

Fig. 3-5

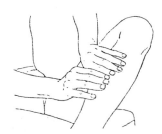

Fig. 3-6

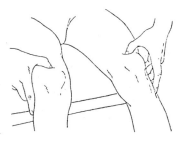

Fig. 3-7

Step 7.
Press Heding (EX-LE 2) with the finger for 10 to 20 times (Fig. 3-7). Indications: myasthenia, arthritis, apoplectic hemiplegia.

Step 8.
Scrub Weizhong (BL 40) on the posterior of the knee for 10 to 20 times (Fig. 3-8). Indications: impotence, lumbago and scelalgia, kidney disease. Also prevents apoplexy.

Step 9.
Grasp the thigh rather heavily from top downward for 10 to 20 times (Fig. 3-9). This promotes blood flow and relaxes muscles of the thigh.

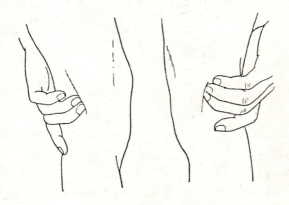

Fig. 3-8

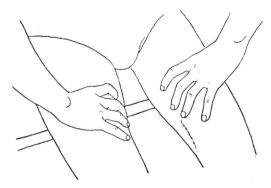

Fig. 3-9

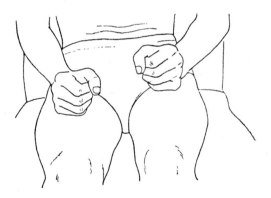

Fig. 3-10

Step 10.
Strike muscles on both thighs with a hollow fist simultaneously, with varying strength and speed (Fig. 3-10). Indications: rheumatism, rheumatoid arthritis. Also prevents apoplectic hemiplegia.

Step 11.
Clap the hip heavily with both hands for 10 to 20 times (Fig. 3-11). Indications: protrusion of intervertebral disc, sciatica, pelvic inflammation, irregular menstruation, impotence, prostatitis, incontinence of urine. Also prevents aseptic necrosis of head of femur, reduces the chance of breaking the femur and tibia for old people.

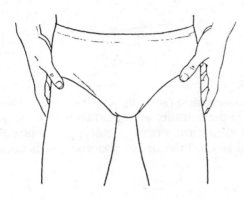

Fig. 3-11

Step 12.
Press each of the two pulsation points of femoral artery with a finger for about one minute, with gradually increasing force until numbness is felt in the toes (Fig. 3-12). Stop pressing. A heat stream will be felt spreading to the legs and feet. This method invigorates the blood flow in the lower limbs, and is indicated in irregular menstruation, Buerger's disease, angitis. Also prevents diseases of the circulatory system in the lower limbs.

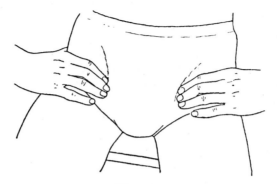

Fig. 3-12

Step 13.

Press Weiwan region (see step 14, Operation 1) with the finger for half a minute, with gradually increasing force (Fig. 3-13). When the pressing is stopped, a heat stream will spread around the upper abdomen. Indication: gastrosis.

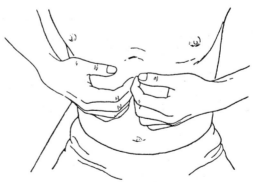

Fig. 3-13

Step 14.
Press Qihai (RN 6) and release repeatedly for 10 to 20 times (Fig. 3-14). Indications: deficiency of *qi* and blood, irregular menstruation.

Step 15.
Rub Qihai (RN 6) with the palm clockwise for 10 to 20 times (Fig. 3-15). Rub the whole abdomen for 20 to 30 times.

Step 16.
Rub rapidly the area between Shangwan (RN 13) and Qugu (RN 2) from top downward with two palms in turn until there is a burning sensation (Fig. 3-16).

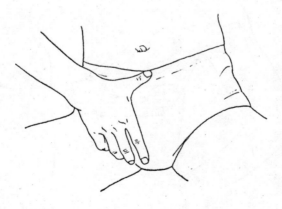

Fig. 3-14

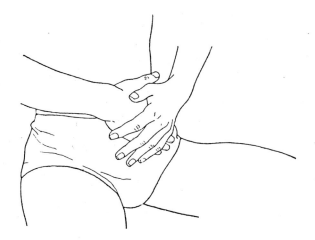

Fig. 3-15

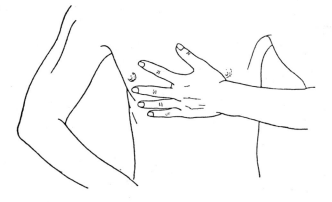

Fig. 3-16

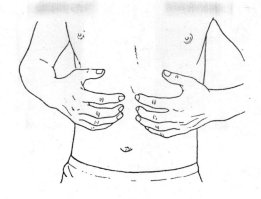

Fig. 3-17

Step 17.
Shape the hands like two paws. Grasp from Shangwan (RN 13) to the sides of the body (Fig. 3-17). Do this repeatedly while slowly moving the action downward to Qugu (RN 2). Do the whole process for 3 to 5 times.

Step 18.
Shape the hands like two paws and scrub from the upper abdomen downward for 3 to 5 times (Fig. 3-18).

Step 19.
Rub the right pectoral muscle with left palm and the left pectoral muscle with right palm in turn for 10 to 20 times (Fig. 3-19).

Step 20.
Tap Danzhong (RN 17) with collected fingertips for 10 to 20 times (Fig. 3-20).

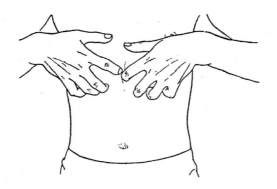

Fig. 3-18

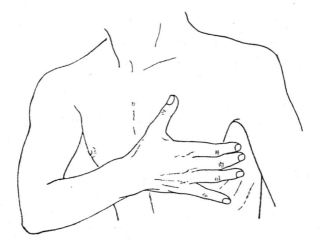

Fig. 3-19

120

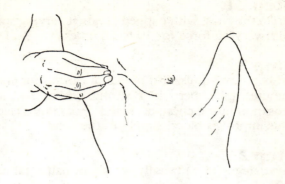

Fig. 3-20

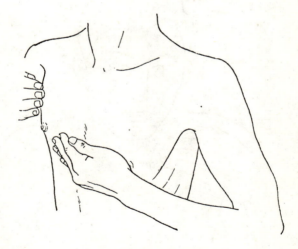

Fig. 3-21

Step 21.
Strike the chest with cupped hands at varying speed and with varying force for 10 to 20 times (Fig. 3-21).

Step 22.
Press the two pulsation points of carotid for about one minute, until there is a strong aching and swelling sensation in the chest, back and upper limbs (Fig. 3-22). This improves blood supply to the head.

Step 23.
Press Hegu (LI 4) heavily for about half a minute (Fig. 3-23).

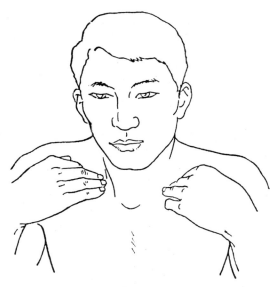

Fig. 3-22

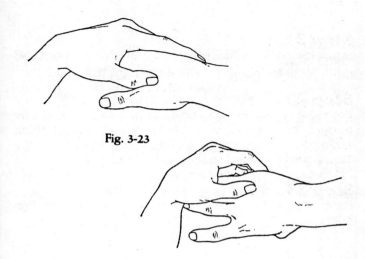

Fig. 3-23

Fig. 3-24

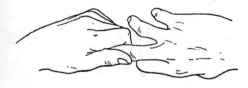

Fig. 3-25

Step 24.
Press and rub Zhongzhu (KI 15) for about half a minute (Fig. 3-24).

Step 25.
Grip the finger at the point where the Sifeng (EX-UE 10) point is located and pull (Fig. 3-25).
Do this to each point on the eight fingers.

Step 26.
Rub rapidly Laogong (PC 8) on the right hand with the thumb of the left hand and rub Laogong (PC 8) on the left hand with the thumb of the right hand for 20 to 30 times (Fig. 3-26). There will be a burning sensation on the palm.

Step 27.
Press Neiguan (PC 6) and Waiguan (SJ 5) on the right hand simultaneously with the left thumb and index

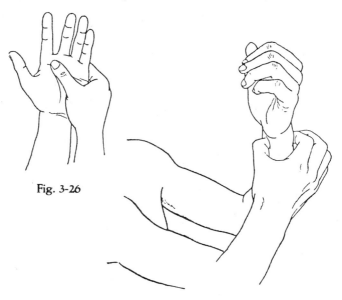

Fig. 3-26

Fig. 3-27

finger, then rub for 10 to 20 times (Fig. 3-27). Do the same to the left hand with the right hand.

Step 28.
Stroke Quchi (LI 11) on the right arm with the thumb of the left hand. Stroke Quchi (LI 11) on the left arm with the thumb of the right hand. (Fig. 3-28)

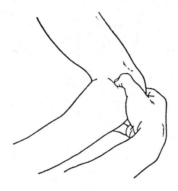

Fig. 3-28

Step 29.
Press and stroke Xiaohai (SI 8) on each arm for 3 to 5 times (Fig. 3-29).

Step 30.
Press and stroke Tianquan (PC 2) on each arm for 3 to 5 times (Fig. 3-30).

Step 31.
Grasp each arm from top downward for 5 to 10 times (Fig. 3-31).

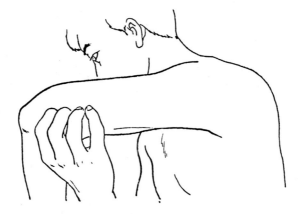

Fig. 3-29

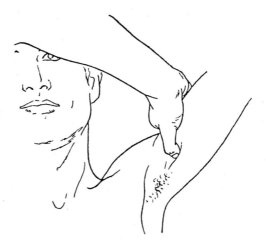

Fig. 3-30

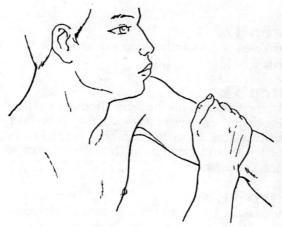

Fig. 3-31

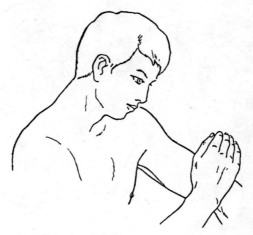

Fig. 3-32

Step 32.
Strike each arm with a cupped hand for 5 to 10 times (Fig. 3-32).

Step 33.
Put the left hand on the right shoulder to steady it, then revolve the right arm forward for 10 to 20 times and backward for 10 to 20 times (Fig. 3-33). Do the same to the left shoulder and arm. This can prevent scapulohumeral periarthritis.

Step 34.
Sit straight, try to stretch the cervical vertebrae upward.

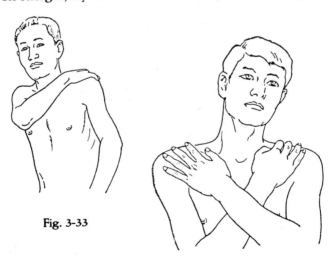

Fig. 3-33

Fig. 3-34

Turn the neck to the left and right for 5 to 10 times (Fig. 3-34). This method indicates hyperosteogeny of the cervical vertebrae, scapulohumeral periarthritis. It is also good for health of the brain.

Step 35.
Press and rub each of the two Taiyang (EX-HN 5) points with a thumb clockwise for 20 to 30 times and counter-clockwise for 20 to 30 times (Fig. 3-35).

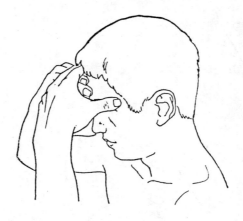

Fig. 3-35

Step 36.
Press the inner canthi with the thumb and index finger (Fig. 3-36).

Step 37.
Pinch the eyebrows for 10 to 20 times (Fig. 3-37).

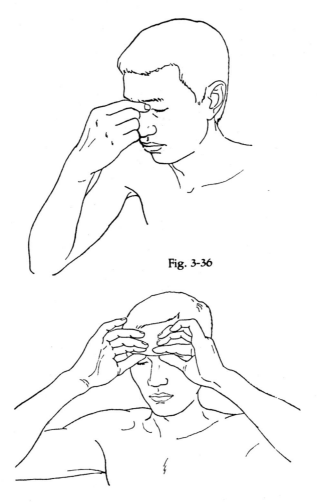

Fig. 3-36

Fig. 3-37

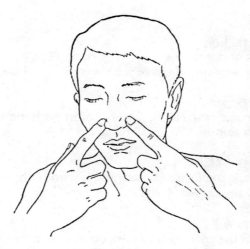

Fig. 3-38

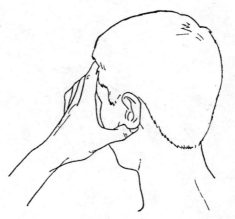

Fig. 3-39

Step 38.
Press and rub the two Yingxiang (LI 20) points with index fingers (Fig. 3-38). Indication: nasal diseases.

Step 39.
Scrub the two Yifeng (SJ 17) points with the thumbs for half a minute (Fig. 3-39).

Step 40.
Massage the face as if washing it with both hands for 10 to 20 times (Fig. 3-40).

Step 41.
Comb the hair with the fingers and thumbs shaped like paws for 10 to 20 times (Fig. 3-41).

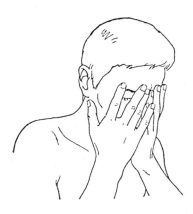

Fig. 3-40

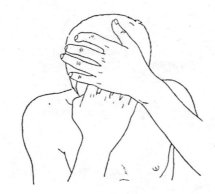

Fig. 3-41

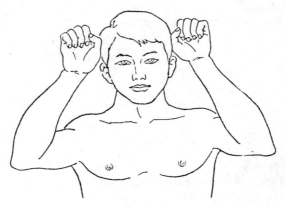

Fig. 3-42

Step 42.
Tap the head with hollow fists for 10 to 20 times (Fig. 3-42).

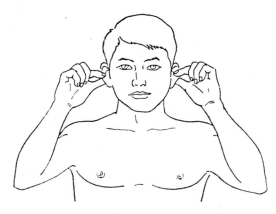

Fig. 3-43

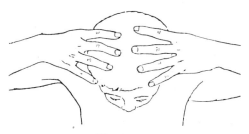

Fig. 3-44

Step 43.
Hold the ear between the thumb and index finger, then rub the ear (Fig. 3-43).

Step 44.
Grasp the scalp with stretched fingers and thumbs bouncingly at varying speed for 10 to 20 times (Fig. 3-44).

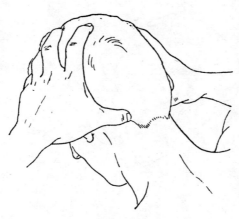

Fig. 3-45

Step 45.
Press and rub the two Fengchi (GB 20) points with the thumbs (Fig. 3-45).

Step 46.
Grasp muscles on the neck for 10 to 20 times (Fig. 3-46).

Step 47.
Grasp muscles on the acromion and Jianjing (GB 21) for 10 to 20 times (Fig. 3-47).

Step 48.
Pinch each side of the waist with a hand for 10 to 20 times (Fig. 3-48).

Step 49.
Pat the whole body with open hands at varying speed and intensity.

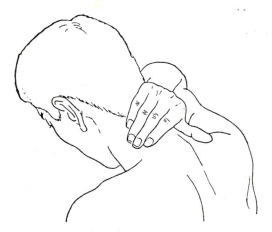

Fig. 3-46

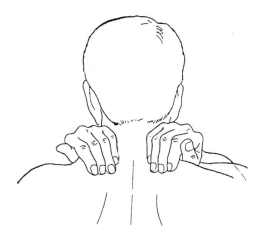

Fig. 3-47

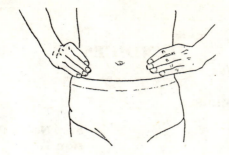

Fig. 3-48

INDICES

For Acupoints:

Point	Step No. in Operation 1
B	
Bafeng (EX-LE 10)	2
Baihui (DU 20)	47
C	
Chengfu (BL 36)	67
Chengjiang (RN 24)	40
Chengqi (ST 1)	39
Chengshan (BL 57)	70
D	
Daheng (SP 15)	22
Danzhong (RN 17)	24
Dazhui (DU 14)	51
Dubi (ST 35)	7
F	
Feishu (BL 13)	58
Fengchi (GB 20)	49
Fengfu (DU 16)	50

Fengshi (GB 31)   11

G

Ganshu (BL 18)   60
Guanyuan (RN 4)   19

H

Heding (EX-LE 2)   8
Hegu (LI 4)   26
Huantiao (GB 30)   66
Huatuojiaji (EX-B 2)   57

J

Jianjing (GB 21)   53
Jiexi (ST 41)   4
Jugu (LI 16)   54

L

Laogong (PC 8)   29

N

Neiguan (PC 6)   30

P

Pishu (BL 20)   61

Q

Qianding (DU 21)   46
Qihai (RN 6)   18
Qihaishu (BL 24)   64

Qihu (ST 13)	23
Quchi (LI 11)	33
Qugu (RN 2)	21

R

Renzhong (DU 26)	41

S

Shangwan (RN 13)	15
Shenshu (BL 23)	63
Sifeng (EX-UE 10)	28
Siqiang (EXTRA)	10
Sizhukong (SJ 23)	44

T

Taichong (LR 3)	3
Taiyang (EX-HN 5)	37
Tianquan (PC 2)	35
Tiantu (RN 22)	25
Tianzong (SI 11)	55
Touwei (ST 8)	43

W

Waiguan (SJ 5)	31
Weishu (BL 21)	62
Weizhong (BL 40)	69

X

Xiaohai (SI 8)	34
Xiawan (RN 10)	17
Ximen (PC 4)	32

Xinshu (BL 15)	59
Xuehai (SP 10)	9

Y

Yanglingquan (GB 34)	6
Yifeng (SJ 17)	45
Yiming (EX-HN 14)	52
Yingxiang (LI 20)	38
Yinmen (BL 37)	68
Yintang (EX-HN 3)	42
Yongquan (KI 1)	71

Z

Zhongji (RN 3)	20
Zhongwan (RN 12)	16
Zhongzhu (KI 15)	27
Zusanli (ST 36)	5

For Indications:

Indication	Step No. in Operation 1

A

abdominal distension	16, 17, 18, 22, 61, 62, 64
amnesia	59
anemia	9, 61
angina pectoris	24, 32, 59
angitis	12
anuresis	21, 67

apoplexy	27, 28, 30, 31, 34, 35, 36, 44, 46, 47
arrhythmia	30, 59
arthralgia of the limbs	33
arthralgia of the neck, shoulder and elbow	34
arthritis, digital	28
arthritis, mandibular	45
arthritis, rheumatic	12
arthritis, rheumatoid	7, 12
arthrosis of the vertebrae	57
asthma	24, 51, 55, 58, 63
asthma, bronchial	25
atrophy, optic	39, 52

B

blepharospasm	39
borborygmi	62, 64
bronchitis	25

C

cerebral anoxia	43
cerebral ischemia	36, 63
cervical spondylopathy	54, 55
chest distress	24
chondromalacia patellae	7
coma	41, 47
common cold	26, 31, 37, 42, 49, 51, 58
constipation	22, 64, 67
coughing	24, 35, 51, 57, 58, 59
coughing with dyspnea	23

D

deafness	31, 45, 63
decrease of vital capacity	23
decreased renal function	67
deficiency of milk secretion	24
diabetes	1
diarrhea	16, 18, 22, 64, 69
diarrhea, chronic	61, 62, 63
disease, kidney	1
disease, knee joint	8
disease, respiratory	57
disease of digestive organs	57
of esophagus	25
of soft tissues	54
of the back	53
of the kidney	66, 69
of the liver and gallbladder	60
of the loin, abdomen and lower limb	57
of the lower limbs and knee joints	69
of the shoulder	53, 58
of the vocal cords	25
diseases, cardiovascular	57
diseases, eye	45, 49
diseases, gastric	14
diseases, gynecological	13
diseases, nasal	38, 42
disorder of the liver-*qi*	3
dysentery	17, 61
dyshormonism	1
dysmenorrhea	9, 18, 19

dyspepsia	16

E

edema	61
encephalopathy	49
enuresis	18, 19
epigastralgia	62
epilepsy	29, 41, 49
excessive sweating	54

F

female sterility	20
fever	51
frequency of micturition	18
fullness in the chest and hypochondrium	23

G

gastralgia	16, 17
gastric dilatation	15
gastric disorder causing nausea	62
gastric ulcer	16
gastritis	15, 16
gastroenteritis, acute	69
gastroptosis	16
gonorrhea	20

H

headaches	3, 4, 37, 42, 43, 44, 47, 49
heart disease	34, 35, 36

heart disease, coronary	27, 29, 31, 41
heart disease, pulmonary	58
heatstroke	29, 41
hematemesis	54, 60
hemiparalysis, facial	39
hemiplegia	26, 49
hemiplegia, apoplectic	10, 13, 33, 67
hemorrhoids	70
hepatitis	61
hiccups	24, 16
hyperosteogeny of the knee joint	7, 69
hypertension	1, 3, 26, 27, 28, 29, 30, 31, 32, 33, 34, 35, 36, 37, 40, 41, 42, 43, 44, 45, 46, 47, 49, 52, 54, 63, 64
hysteria	30

I

impotence	13, 18, 19, 21, 63, 64, 69
indigestion	61, 62
infection, urinary tract	63
influenza	44
insomnia	29, 42, 50, 52
irregular menstruation	2, 3, 9, 18, 19, 63

L

laryngopharyngitis	25
leukorrhagia	20
leukorrhea, morbid	21, 63

lumbago	11, 33, 64, 66, 68, 69, 70
lumbago, chronic	63

M

malnutrition and indigestion in children	28
mastitis	3, 32, 53
measles	33
migraine	31
myasthenia	11
myasthenia, general	51
myasthenia of the lower limbs	4, 8, 10, 67
myopia	39

N

nausea	30
neuralgia, intercostal	24
neurasthenia	26, 59
neuritis, peripheral	2
night sweating	58

O

obstruction, acute gastric	16
obstruction, urethral	20
obstruction, urinary	69

P

pain, abdominal	5, 19, 26, 64, 69
pain, back	33, 60, 61, 63, 68
pain, chest	23, 24

pain, hypochondriac	60
pain, lumbosacral	13, 67
pain of the dorsum of the foot, swelling	2
pain in the arm	54
pain in the chest and hypochondrium	30, 62
pain in the knee joint	6
pain in the leg	11, 66, 70
pain in the vertebral column	60
palpitation due to fright	59
palsy, brachial	34, 35, 36, 55
palsy of the hand	26
paralysis	8, 47, 66, 70
paralysis, apoplectic	12, 32, 54, 55
paralysis, facial	26, 37, 38, 40, 44, 45
paralysis of the lower limbs	5, 6, 11, 13, 67, 68
paraparesis	66
parotitis	45
pertussis	28
pheumonia	31
pleurisy	32
prolapse of the anus	47, 70
prolapse of the uterus	19, 20, 47
prostatitis	18
pruritus vulvae	19
psychosis	29, 41, 47, 50
psychosis, manic-depressive	51
pyrexia	33

R

respiratory failure	41

retention of urine	18, 63
rheumarthritis	4
rheumatism	7
rhinitis	49

S

scapulohumeral periarthritis	54, 55
scelalgia caused by protrusion of intervertebral disc	13
sciatica	13, 66, 67, 68, 69, 70
seminal emission	13, 18, 63, 69
sequelae of apoplexy	50
shock	30, 41
sore throat	30
spasm, facial	38
spasm of cardia of stomach	15
spasm of diaphragm	25
spasm of leg muscles	70
stasis of blood flow	12
stiffness and pain of nape	49, 51
stiffness of the back	51
stomachache	30, 57, 60,
stomatitis	29
strabismus	44
suffocation	41

T

tachycardia	32, 59
thyroid enlargement	25
tinnitus	45, 49, 52, 63
tonsillitis	26
toothaches	26, 45

trigeminal neuralgia	37, 38, 39, 40
tuberculosis, lymphoid	54

U

uterine bleeding	3
uterine bleeding, dysfunctional	9

V

vertigo	3, 42, 43, 47, 49, 52
vexation	59
vomiting	16, 17, 29, 61, 62, 69
vomiting, neurogenic	25

W

weakness of kidney-*qi*	63
weakness of the heart	23
weakness of the spleen and the stomach	61, 62

图书在版编目(CIP)数据

中医按摩健身操:英文/陈兆广编著.
—北京:外文出版社,1992(1997重印)
ISBN 7-119-01480-3

Ⅰ.中… Ⅱ.陈… Ⅲ.按摩-保健操-英文 Ⅳ.R161

中国版本图书馆 CIP 数据核字(96)第 19752 号

责任编辑 陈有升
封面设计 朱振安

中医按摩健身操
陈兆广编著

*

ⓒ外文出版社
外文出版社出版
(中国北京百万庄大街24号)
邮政编码 100037
北京外文印刷厂印刷
中国国际图书贸易总公司发行
(中国北京车公庄西路35号)
北京邮政信箱第399号 邮政编码100044
1992年(34开)第1版
1997年第1版第2次印刷
(英)
ISBN 7-119-01480-3/R·84(外)
00950
14-E-2727P